THE OPIOID EPIDEMIC OF AMERICA:

WHAT YOU NEED KNOW ABOUT THE OPIATE AND OPIOID CRISIS... AND HOW WE CAN HEAL FROM IT

By D.W. Graeme

The Opioid Epidemic Of America:
What You Need Know About The Opiate and Opioid Crisis... And How We Can Heal From It

TABLE OF CONTENTS

THE OPIOID EPIDEMIC OF AMERICA: INTRODUCTION .8

CHAPTER 1:
THE OPIATE ADDICTION EPIDEMIC 13

CHAPTER 2:
DEFINITION OF OPIATES & THEIR HISTORY 19

    OPIATES THROUGHOUT HISTORY 20

CHAPTER 3: HOW OPIATES WORK 24

    PAIN'S RE-CLASSIFICATION 26
    WHY DO PEOPLE GET ADDICTED TO OPIATES? 27
    WHAT FACTORS LEAD TO ADDICTION? 27
    HARD TO MEASURE HONESTLY 30
    OXYS SAVES THE DAY? 34
    OXYCONTIN, OXYCODONE &
    WHERE WE ARE NOW 35
    THE SHORTCOMINGS OF OXYCONTIN 39
    A TRAGIC "PRESCRIPTION" 40
    THE SLIPPERY SLOPE 43

CHAPTER 4:
TROUBLING ABUSE AMONG TEENAGERS 50

SIGNS AND SYMPTOMS 51

WHAT CAN YOU DO AS A PARENT? 52

TEEN PRESCRIPTION DRUG ABUSE PREVENTION 54

HOW WE CAN HEAL 57

CHAPTER 5:
TECHNIQUES TO OVERCOME OPIOID ADDICTION...
ONCE AND FOR ALL 58

Detox Treatment Help 58

Over-the-Counter Cures 59

Taper Technique 60

Buprenorphine......................................60

Changes in Daily Routine 61

Attending Support Groups.......................61

Psychotherapy 62

Residential Treatment Programs.............62

Outpatient Treatment Programs.............64

Individual Treatment Needs 65

CHAPTER 6:
YOUR SUPPORT SYSTEM
& GETTING REAL...67

CHAPTER 7:
CHOICES FOR DETOXING 72

MEDICATIONS THAT CAN BEAT
OPIOID ADDICTION 74

CHAPTER 8:
GETTING READY FOR DETOX................................79

CHAPTER 9:
WITHDRAWAL SYMPTOMS.........................85

COPING & WITHDRAWAL SYMPTOMS 88
HOME REMEDIES FOR COPING
WITH WITHDRAWAL SYMPTOMS.................................88
OVER-THE-COUNTER HELP 89
STAY SAFE AND COMFORTABLE 90
TREATING WITHDRAWAL..91

CHAPTER 10:
HOW TO STAY CLEAN 93

GOALS CAN MAKE A DIFFERENCE 102
WHAT TO DO IF YOU RELAPSE 104
COPING WITH PRESCRIPTION DRUG ABUSE...................106

HELPING A FAMILY MEMBER OR FRIEND 108
INTERVENTION 110
PREVENTING PRESCRIPTION DRUG ABUSE 110

CHAPTER 11:
CONCLUSION 113

The Opioid Epidemic of America: Introduction

America's opioid crisis and opiate addiction is ever-changing and has a lot to do with market conditions. Supply and demand along with basic economics play a greater role than many people realize in which drugs come in and out of fashion at a particular point in time. Regardless of which form of opioids are popular at the present moment, there is little doubt that opiates will always be one of the most widely abused classes of drugs.

Whether it be Vicodin, Oxys, Fentanyl, Methadone or Heroin, the opiate addict will generally take what they can get their hands on and then abuse the hell out of it.

And, unfortunately, the results are often deadly.

There are over 52,000 drug overdose deaths per year in the United States, 65 percent of which are opioid-related.

That means that 92 people every single day die from an opioid overdose.

Opiates are natural drugs derived from opium while as opioids are drugs that act like opiates, however are synthetic or semi-synthetic drugs. For the sake of this book, we will use the terms opioids and opiates interchangeably.

See, opiates have a very long and rich history of being "in fashion", later shunned by society and then again, finding their medicinal use for the management of pain.

It was this last rise however, in the use of prescription opiate painkillers prescribed by doctors and pushed by Big Pharma, that has brought about what the CDC is now calling an epidemic of prescription drug addiction. In fact, in 2017 nearly 3.1 million Americans were addicted to some form of prescription painkiller, more than those addicted to cocaine and heroin combined.

I have been clean from my opiate addiction for over 13 years, yet the memory of the day to day struggle, the terror and hopelessness, are still fresh in my mind. This is not something that I expect to ever forget and it was interesting to re-live some of it and learn a few new "tricks" and strategies in the writing of this book.

What scares the hell out of me more than anything else is the rising problem, in epidemic proportions, of heroin use in this country as a direct result of prescription opiate addiction. There is no doubt that prescription painkillers serve as a gateway to heroin use and this is deadly.

While abuse of prescription pills for pain was reported to be going down in 2011, according to the national survey on drug use and health, heroin use was reported to be increasing. In fact, in 2011, nearly 200,000 people tried heroin for the first time. By 2017, the rates for prescription drug abuse were back up into the stratosphere and heroin abuse nearly out of control, with an estimate of over 700,000 Americans having used the drug.

If you or a loved one have an Opioid or Opiate addiction, or you want insights on this epidemic, this book is for you.

In this Book, you will learn more about this epidemic, the tipping point for opioid drugs, their effects on your body and mind. Finally, I cover what you can do to break free.

There is also information on opiate maintenance programs as well as warnings on their long-term use. I have included some good information about opiate detox and making treatment decisions if necessary.

Recovery from opiate addiction isn't easy but it is absolutely possible and I have found that it is infinitely simpler and more fulfilling than that of the day to day life of a hopeless opioid addict.

Lastly, it can be said that there is a group of people using opioids in their lives to manage their pain, where this is the only solution to the pain. Hopefully this book can help you see ways to improve your life and dependency on these addictive opioids.

Take what you can from this, and if you can, help another. Thank you for taking this journey with me.

- D.W. Graeme

Chapter 1: The Opiate Addiction Epidemic

Most people think that they have a clear picture in their mind of what a drug addict is but generally, when it comes to opiate addiction, you get couldn't be further from that image.

Opiate addicts do not fit a general stereotype as the drug does not discriminate.

Old, young, short, tall, healthy, smart, sick. It doesn't matter.

Because of the nature of opiate addiction, it strikes across age, ethnic and economic groups and then pulls each and every one of those stricken down with equal measure.

A recent report by the CDC discussed how America's opioid addiction is now the fastest growing drug problem we have to deal with. The total number of painkillers prescribed in a just single year is enough to medicate every single adult living in the U.S., around the clock!

In fact, more people are killed by drug overdoses - most of them resulting from opioid use - than guns or car accidents!

While it is true that heroin is the most widely used illegal opiate, it's a fact that prescription opioid / opiate painkillers are both dangerous as well as an insidious problem in our healthcare system. The World Health Organization (WHO) estimates that approximately over three million people in the United States alone are addicted to prescription opiates.

The problem is also not limited to adults, as first use of opiates seems to be getting younger. A report by the

National Institute on Drug Abuse (NIDA) reported an estimated 52+ million people, 20% of those from the ages of 12 and up, have used, at least once, prescription drugs for non-medical reasons. Also, about 1 in 12 high school seniors reported non-medical use of the prescription drug Vicodin during the past year. About 1 in 20 high school seniors also reported abusing OxyContin. This isn't limited to the younger crowd either.

According to a 2011 study by the Substance Abuse and Mental Health Services Administration (SAMHSA), the rate of current illicit drug use in adults aged 50 to 59 increased to 6.3% in 2011 from 2.7% in 2002 with opiates being among the most commonly abused drugs.

The total number of opiate prescriptions dispensed by retail pharmacies in the United States rose from 76 million in 1991 to 526 million in 2017.

This great epidemic of unprecedented opiate addictions and painkiller addictions results in nearly 33,000 overdose deaths annually. While heroin continues to be a rising problem, opiate addiction, in general, is not the stereotypical drug problem that many of us think of when we picture the "war on drugs."

In fact, many times this involves a patient who began with a legitimate pain issue, an unwitting string of physicians (or not) who are writing these prescriptions, and pharmaceutical companies who are (debatably) acting within the law. The public consumption of opiates, through legal channels, is costing health insurers over $72 billion annually.

Opiates are a huge problem....and growing. Trust me, I know.

Most of the time, we start taking the opioids for a legitimate pain issue, whether for a root canal or some major surgery.

Many times though, the addiction from the opiate can develop over a period of time as a physical dependency. With others, however, there is an instantaneous "pull" that these drugs have on you because of the way that they make you feel. They not only take away the physical pain that they were prescribed for, but bring to the table something that you thought you had been looking for for a very long time. This is how it was for me. Those pills became my best friend and my salvation for a time - until they completely owned me.

You will find peace not by trying to escape your problems, but by confronting them courageously. You will find peace not in denial, but in victory.

-J. Donald Walters

Chapter 2: Definition of Opiates & Their History

Opium teaches only one thing,
which is that aside from physical
suffering,
there is nothing real.
- Andre Malraux

Opiates, by definition, are considered "to be the natural alkaloids found in the resin of the opium poppy (Papaver somniferum)."

However, some definitions of opiates include the semi-synthetic substances that are derived directly from the opium poppy as well. As such, opiates themselves can be natural or synthetic. Natural opiates include opium, morphine, and codeine. Other substances that are man-made are called opioids. These are most used to treat chronic pain and are also highly addictive. These include Methadone, Vicodin, Oxycodone, Demerol, and Dilaudid. Heroin is actually an opioid manufactured from morphine.

Opiates Throughout History

While opiate addiction is at the forefront of the news and wreaking havoc in so many lives in the present day, it is by no means a new phenomenon.

In fact, the first opiates were believed to have been cultivated and used during the Neolithic period (the new stone age). The Sumerian, Egyptian, Greek, Roman, Persian and Arab Empires all used opiates as a potent pain relief measure, even allowing for prolonged surgical procedures.

The first written reference to the poppy used to produce opium appears in a Sumerian text dated around 4,000 B.C.

The great Homer also speaks of its' effects in The Odyssey. In this part of the story, Telemachusis depressed after failing to find his father, Odysseus. But then Helen...

"...had a happy thought. Into the bowl in which their wine was mixed, she slipped a drug that had the power of robbing grief and anger of their sting and banishing all painful memories. No one who swallowed this dissolved in their wine could shed a single tear that day, even for the death of his mother or father, or if they put his brother or his own son to the sword and he were there to see it done..."

Images of poppies appear in Egyptian pictography and Roman sculptures. Representations of the Greek and Roman gods of sleep, Hypnos and Somnos, often show them wearing or carrying poppies. Opium was readily bought on the streets of Rome. Opium use had spread to India, China, and Arabia by the eighth century A.D. Arabs both used opium and organized its trade.

In China, recreational use of the drug began in the 15th century and increased to near epidemic levels until the 17th century, when opium prohibition began there. This followed another two centuries of increased opium use and several trade "opium-related" wars. By 1905, nearly 25% of the male population of China were regular opium users.

British opium imports rose from a brisk 91,000 lbs in 1830 to an astonishing 280,000 lbs in 1860. With the invention of the hypodermic syringe during the mid-nineteenth century, the use of injectable painkillers, including morphine, during the American Civil War is what formed the first wave in America of morphine addiction.

However, one of the most important reasons for this increase in opiate consumption within the United States, specifically during the 19th century, was the heavy prescribing as well as dispensing of legal opiates by pharmacists and physicians to women with "female problems" (mostly to relieve menstrual pain). Between 150,000 and 200,000 opiate addicts lived in the United States in the late 19th century and between two-thirds and three-quarters of these addicts were women.

Chapter 3:
How Opiates Work

Whether you sniff it smoke it eat it or shove it up your ass, the result is the same: addiction.
-William S. Burroughs

As opioid addiction has become front page news everywhere or may even be very prevalent in your life, it is important to understand exactly how opiates work. This will help us better understand how to treat and heal from it.

Opiate addiction is often characterized by a noted increase in the tolerance for the particular drug used and, if the person also has pain issues, a revisit of the original issues and symptoms. This is an absolutely maddening cycle. I know because I lived it.

I began taking Vicodin in my early thirties for some moderate neck pain. I became immediately addicted because I loved the pills and the feeling they gave me.

What I found, though, was that I needed to take more and more of them to get the desired effect. So much so that, in the end, I was taking over 30 pills a day and I could have taken a lot more had I had access to them. Through most of this, I wasn't taking the pills for fun anymore. It was only "fun" in the very beginning when I was being enticed and romanced by the drug.

No, I was only taking them to feel "normal" and avoid getting sick. This was a horrific way to live but painkiller addiction is powerful.

Drugs are a bet with your mind.
-Jim Morrison

13

Pain's Re-Classification

Opiates produce euphoria or a sense of well-being in human beings which can make them addicted to them. Legally, opiates are used to treat body pain. When they are used as pain relievers however, people tend to develop tolerance, an increased desire for these drugs.

It means that they need relatively heavier doses of these drugs in comparison to what they used earlier, to get relief from pain. Continuous usage of opiates for a specific period of time may cause obsession or addiction in some people. These people start to obsessively think how to get more opiates. In most of the cases, they get engaged in illegitimate activities, such as double doctoring, where someone "shops" doctors to get larger amounts of opioids than would normally be administered by one single physician.

Why do people get addicted to opiates?

A heavy dose of opiates may cause death due to respiratory or cardiac arrest. The reason why people increase the intake of these drugs is because of the difference between tolerance to euphoric and dangerous effect. Opiates develop tolerance to the euphoric effects faster than rather dangerous effects. Because of this phenomenon, people often overdose unintentionally to accomplish their desires or relieve from pain.

Some, like my cousin, struggled with the increasing urges to use cocaine and other harder drugs. He unfortunately, in the end, died of an overdose. A father's life cut down in his prime.

What factors lead to addiction?

While medical experts are still looking for answers to find the exact cause of addiction to these drugs, a general perception says that an addiction of anything is actually the product of many factors.

These factors are:

- **Psychological:** Majority of opiate addicts belong to the people who have a mindset to self-medicate health issues, particularly anxiety, tension, depression and headaches. Mental illness may also indicate a person's potential to addiction.
- **Biological:** According to medical research, individuals with a lack of the neurotransmitter, called "endorphins", try to self-medicate this birth deficiency. In their attempts of maintain the level of neurotransmitters, they may take opiates, such as opium and get into trouble.
- **Environmental:** People who are surrounded by addicts or have a disordered home

environment are likely to get addicted at any point of life.

- *Genetic:* People who have blood relative with addiction disorder have a high chance of becoming opiate addicts. However, there are quite a few individuals who still live unaffected with addicted parents or siblings.

- *Accidental:* Many individuals have reported they became opiate addicts while going through prolonged post-accident opiate medication period.

The fire of opiate addiction was already burning even before pills such as Oxycontin existed, but this one pill, which can be argued, has single handedly transformed this smaller crisis into a nationwide epidemic.

The Center for Disease Control has called the current overdose epidemic the "worst drug overdose epidemic in [U.S.] history".

17

Prescription drug abuse is an issue that touches nearly everybody in this nation. Doctors over-prescribe in order to help patients or possible some for profit.

This issue has reared its head from time to time, but prior to 1990s pain medication was not nearly as severe of a problem.

What exactly could have happened to spark such a drastic change?

Hard To Measure Honestly

Amongst a few other things, implementation of pain indicators contributed to this change in pain killer addiction.

See, there were originally only four vital indicators that doctors used to diagnose patients, but eventually pain became the fifth one.

Heart rate, blood pressure, body temperature, and breathing rate were the original four signs. All of these four signs are measured or observed during a routine check-up.

Eventually, however, pain was re-classified as a "Fifth" indicator, although it cannot be measured as easily. Anecdotal evidence from doctors reports suggests that many of them may have disagreed with this re-classification.

With the original four indicators, they were fairly easy to measure or at least observe. Pain is not as easy to observe, but doctors have done their best to try.

Patients are typically asked to rate their pain on a scale of 1 to 10 to determine what their needs are. You may have seen one of these charts yourself if you have been to a clinic or ER lately.

It can be an effective tool if you are honest and use it to get the dose you need, but anybody with addictive tendencies can easily game the system.

Pain can be hard to measure anyways, and chronic pain has the potential to be quite debilitating, so it is not something that can be ignored. However, it seems that making it a fifth vital indicator may not have been the best solution.

That major shift in the way pain was classified treated is what allowed the explosion of Oxycontin.

Skeptical Scalpel, a popular medical blogger who is a retired Physician, explains exactly why pain can be hard to treat.

"Despite efforts to quantify it with numbers and scales using smiley and frown faces, it is highly subjective. Pain is a symptom. Pain is not a vital sign, nor is it a disease."

When pain management became a big issue, doctors were now told to use pain as a way to diagnose a patient. Unfortunately, it is difficult to accurately measure levels of pain, no matter how real they are.

Because of this, a "drug seeking" person now had a motivation to fabricate the level of their pain.

Doctors have become so used to this drug seeking behavior, that they have become more likely to assume somebody is seeking drugs, even if they are not. They have found it hard to discern the true needs for pain relief among the many who abuse the system.

In 1985, the World Health Organization began encouraging doctors to prescribe opioid pain killers such as Percocet for long term cancer pain.

Before that, these medications were typically used for short term pain. The result was that now companies had a reason to try and create a new formula, that combined the short and long term pain relief benefits.

This revised new and improved formula of pills would have dire consequences for millions of unsuspecting patients, and paved the way for main management to become a big business.

Let's look at what happens when doctors are pressured to over-prescribe, and when they are given a dangerous drug to dispense by greedy pharmaceutical companies.

When Oxycodone and more specifically Oxycontin was released, it completely changed the face of painkiller addiction.

Oxys Saves the Day?

Before we learn about Purdue Pharmaceuticals, the company at the heart of this scandal, we need to understand the pill they pushed: Oxycontin.

Governor Peter Shumlin of Vermont stated that Oxycontin *"lit the match that ignited America's opiate and heroin crisis"* and called for a limit in the number of pills that can be included in a prescription.

I was very familiar with Oxycontin as a street drug user, even though I was mostly just did pot then. You could say I was fortunate in that regard, and I never actually did Oxycontin.

By the mid 2000s and the drug had already sunk its teeth into many other people and culture. It was even glamorized in a song I used to listen to when I was in high school, called "Oxy Cotton" from a rapper named "Lil Wyte".

Songs like that only added to the drug's allure and fueled it's spread across America.

Oxycontin, Oxycodone & Where We Are Now

The names Oxycontin and Oxycodone describe separate pills, and we will examine the differences between the two and how they could have caused so much damage.

For those of you who have been through your own personal ringer with pills, you are likely familiar with Oxycontin. I think it is important to understand just what Oxycodone is, because it is the main chemical in this dangerous class of pills.

Oxycodone itself is the opioid that Oxycontin is derived from, and it was first created in Germany. It wasn't created in some mad scientist's lab that wanted to take over the world, it was just meant to be a superior painkiller to those that currently existed.

Oxycodone first came to the U.S. in 1939, however it took a while for it be used widely and adopted. That is until 1996, when Purdue Pharmaceuticals began manufacturing it in it's new tablet form, Oxycontin.

24

By 2001 it was the most widely used painkiller, and was beginning to be abused by many people.

It came in two forms, the extended release, and the fast release. Between these two, Oxycodone would also typically be mixed with aspirin or Tylenol as well which produced many different versions.

The extended release form was known as OxyContin, and was also one of the more widely used iterations of this drug.

In theory, it worked perfectly. It was designed to deliver the dose of painkiller needed over the course of 12 hours, so a patient would not have to constantly be taking pills. However, it was only theory.

There are plenty of legitimate patients that have benefited from this type of medication, but they also carried a high potential for abuse, especially before their reformulation in 2010.

Purdue Pharmaceuticals, the company that manufactured Oxycontin, touted it as the solution for patients with long-term pain.

Instead of having to wake up in the middle of the night to take another dose, it would allow for pain relief over long periods such as an 8 hour sleep cycle.

This is actually a very real phenomenon because I remember my grandma having to be visited in the middle of the night for her next dose of Hydrocodone.

Of course prescribing Oxycontin was usually still over-kill even as an extended release. Oxycontin was not the only way Oxycodone was packaged, and it also came in fast release formulas.

The quick release form was typically called Roxycodone or "Roxys" but also could be found under names such as OxyFast or OxyIR.

These fast release forms had the most potential for abuse, because they produced the instant euphoria a drug addict seeks.

The Shortcomings of Oxycontin

Despite how promising Oxycontin sounded, it was not nearly as effective or safe as physicians were originally made to believe. Studies from Medical Professionals and complaints from patients quickly began to surface, indicating that Oxycontin had many shortcomings.

In 2001, The Medical Letter on Drugs and Therapeutics concluded that "Oxycodone offered no advantage over appropriate doses of other potent opioids. "

Their medicine was not viable for marketing as short term pain relief, as superior short term pain medicines were already widely used by then.

Research shows that the stronger the dose, the greater the health risks of Oxycodone, and it also increases risk for overdose. This only added fuel to the fire, as more medicine was used to make up for not lasting the intended duration.

Currently, over half of all long-term Oxycontin users are on doses considered dangerously high by public health officials. That is a strong call to action. This was based on a report conducted for the LA Times, using an analysis of nationwide prescription data.

Since Oxycontin is still an opiate, albeit a synthetic one, it carries the same risk for dependence, abuse and withdrawal that Heroin does. In fact it was nicknamed "Hillbilly Heroin" by some users in the Midwest.

A Tragic "Prescription"

LAPD officer Ernest Gallego's story demonstrates just how dangerous Oxycontin is.

According to his family, he was placed on the drug after a back injury he sustained in a major car accident. After the accident, which was life changing, he was immediately prescribed Oxycontin.

Since the injury was major, he experienced chronic pain and had a reason to need pain relief. Eventually he began to display the typical signs of opiate abuse. Fender-benders and grogginess became common, and his family tried to cut off his prescription.

He thought he had it under control, and I can't blame him for thinking that. I always said that same thing with my drug problem, but to be honest, I was wrong.

Soon he was found lying forward on his steering wheel, and was taken to the hospital. The next day he fell asleep at his father's home, and never woke up.

The coroner's report showed that he had lethal levels of Oxycontin in his system, and his prescription bottle showed that he had 1/5th the amount left that he should have.

This man was a police officer and a hero, so his strong moral fiber was not the main cause of his inability to control his prescription drugs. I know he never intended to end up in such a bad situation, but once a drug problem has progressed to that stage, it can be very hard to fix it.

This tragic example illustrates how even somebody with chronic pain can end up losing their life to the pill that was supposed to help them.

Again, there are exceptions to this where this is the ONLY solution in order to survive the agony of the pain that is experiences without them.

However, like all opioids, Oxycontin had a major potential for abuse, but Purdue downplayed it as long as they could.

The Slippery Slope

I met many men and women in drug rehab who were there solely for prescription drug abuse, where Oxycontin and Hydrocodone were usually the culprits.

Patients whose medication wears off early can suffer both a return of their underlying pain and as well as the starting stages of strong withdrawal symptoms. This is often a large motivator for people to take even more drugs to counter-balance the effect.

Opioid users risk increasing tolerance over time. This leads to less pain relief, as well as a withdrawal symptoms becoming more likely to occur.

This also leads to doctors having to prescribe higher doses to patients in order to combat the higher tolerance for the drug, and raising the dosage raises the stakes, as well as the potential consequences.

I am all to familiar with these higher highs, and lower lows leading somebody into a downward spiral that can be hard to break out of. I have experienced opiate detox, and I would not wish it on my worst enemy.

For now, it is important to note that the risks of over-prescribing opioids were obvious, even early on. It turns out that many patients seeking pain relief ended up in a different kind of pain.... the pain of an opioid addiction.

The addictive centers of the brain are very risky to poke at, and at the time, Oxycontin was the perfect drug to get people hooked who may not have even had addictive tendencies.

Addiction is a complex brain disorder, but based on my own experience I can say that certain people like me are pre-disposed. I was engaging in addictive behavior and thinking patterns well before I ever smoked pot, and I have met many addicts with similar stories.

However, I have also met many people with drug problems that were clearly not predestined for drug addiction. Their addiction had instead been sparked by the powerful effects of painkillers like Oxycontin and Vicodin.

In rehab, it was common to see an ordinary person who was often much older than the typical drug addict. They were often not engaging in illegal behavior, and have merely ran into problems due to prescription painkillers, and had to resort to treatment.

Oxycontin was also easy to tamper with when addicts first discovered it, so even in though it was an extended release, it could still be abused. I knew of all this without ever touching the drug, because I used to be fascinated by documentaries on the subject.

The knowledge of how easy it was to abuse Oxycontin was so widespread that it only added to the allure the drug's name carried for drug users.

The coating was not so secure at first, and users were able to easily remove it which allowed them to break down and inject the pill, or snort it for immediate effects.

Injecting drugs greatly increases the risk for overdose, and increases the harm done to the user in many different ways.

I have nothing against somebody getting relief for their pain, but clearly there was a negligence here in that these pills had many known risks. They were being prescribed for much lower levels of pain than their strength warranted, and carried too high levels of abuse to be justified.

Oxycodone has been re-formulated and mixed with Naltrexone, which blocks the euphoric effects of opiates. This is a very recent development meant to stem the tide of abuse, but too much damage has already been done.

The new security features on the pills that have been introduced recently have made it much harder to abuse Oxycontin. This would seem like a good thing, but most people were already hooked by now.

The fact that it is harder to abuse now, has actually backfired, and led to an increase in the abuse of street drugs like heroin.

Another important fact of Oxycontin on the streets, is the high price tag it carries.

There is no way to measure it exactly, as street drug prices vary, but I have heard stories of it costing 1$ per milligram. For an addict that has developed a habit, it seems like 40-80mg is required, but many will require more than 100mg after a tolerance is built up.

This is compared to street heroin, which is usually about 20-40$ for a similar high. Many users have voluntarily switched to street drugs to save money. This is a sad fact.

In hard hit areas such as the Northeast, these pills can still fetch a high bounty.

A movie called "Oxymorons" illustrated just how coveted the powerful opiates were. It tells the true story of a group of young men that robbed a Boston pharmacy for Oxycontin, and ended up with drastic consequences.

This high price tag on Oxycontin has also led to all sorts of greed. Still, this high street demand made it attractive for drug users and profiteers to find a good source and redistribute them illegally.

Unfortunately the real cause of Oxycontin's rise, and the subsequent rise in it's street value, can be traced back to one company and how it decided to market it's double-edged sword of a painkiller.

According to the federal government's National Survey on Drug

Use and Health, more than 8 million Americans have abused OxyContin over the last 20 years.

That's too high. We can turn this tide.

Chapter 4: Troubling Abuse Among Teenagers

Every day, there are a lot of teens who are using prescription drugs without any guidance from a doctor. Many of them are doing this for the first time, and some, are using drugs for non-medical purposes. According to a survey done by Monitoring the Future in 2015, prescription drugs and OTCs are the most regularly abused drugs by 12th graders. Next in line is marijuana, alcohol, and tobacco.

Most of the teens and young adults have access to prescription drugs through their friends and relatives. They get these drugs without the knowledge of others because the drugs are readily seen and available at home and from friends' parents medicine cabinets.

Prescription drug abuse among teens stems from their desire to get the feeling of soaring, to treat pain, and sometimes they believe that it will make them perform better in class. Boys are usually inclined to abuse drugs to get high. Girls usually do it to lose weight and remain alert.

Signs and Symptoms

If you are a parent, then it is important to know and be aware of the signs as well as possible symptoms of prescription drug abuse, so you can immediately take action if your child suffers from it.

Some of the most common are as follows:

- Irregular schedule

- Changes in circles of friends

- Lack of interest in appearance, sports, and social activities

- Missing cash and valuables at home

- Sudden changes in mood

- Being secretive

- Increase in snoring

What can you do as a parent?

As busy as parents can be, it is vital to take notice of your child's performance in school and other activities.

Stay up-to-date and show your child that you care, by asking how his or her day went.

Doing this every day can help you notice if there are any changes in your child's behavior, especially if he or she is in the teenage years.

Here are some helpful tips for parents:

- Educate yourself and know the possible signs and symptoms of prescription drug abuse among teenagers.

- Increase awareness of your child's behavior and activities.

- Keep your medications in a safe place. Lock it if necessary.

- Monitor your medication so that you will know if a pill or two is missing.

- If you have any unused medication then make sure to properly dispose of them.

- Get to know the friends of your teenager. Find time to bond with him or her and see what the conversations are about.

- Monitor online activity: To monitor or not to monitor? This decision lies entirely on the parents. Today, the internet is very accessible to all ages as long as you have a computer and an internet connection. Kids sometimes get past parental controls as they sometimes prove to be more tech-savvy than their parents.

As a parent, you need to know that prescription medications can easily be obtained online from both legitimate and rogue online pharmacies.

The majority of the online pharmacies are operating illegally and they do not have a pharmacist. There are also a lot of counterfeit drugs and if your child gets a hold of these, there is no way of knowing the end results may be.

Teen Prescription Drug Abuse Prevention

Young people are at a relatively high risk for prescription drug abuse as compared to adults. Here are steps that you can follow to prevent it from happening:

- **Make sure to stress the dangers of prescription drug abuse to your teenage child.** Let him/her know that even though it is prescribed by a doctor, it does not mean that anyone can take it. This is very important especially if your child has other current prescription medications.

- **Have rules for prescription drugs.** Let your child know that sharing the prescription medication is a big no-no. It is illegal. Emphasize the weight of taking the dose as instructed by the doctor. Let your child know that he or she cannot make changes to the prescription.

- **Dispose of the medications in your home properly.** Do not flush the drugs in the toilet unless your pharmacist says so. The local trash service may have a provision that accepts unopened or unused medications. If you are going to throw unused medicines in your trash at home, you should remove them from the container and mix them with coffee grounds, along with some other unwanted substances. As for the container, remove and destroy the label before throwing it out.

How We Can Heal

Chapter 5: Techniques to overcome opioid addiction... Once and for all

Detox Treatment Help

This is the first step to treating opiate addiction. This is the removal of drugs from the system of an addict.

For most people, withdrawal effects of opiates keep them from taking the very first steps towards living a drug-free life. Detox programs offer psychological as well as the physical support that a person requires in order to stop utilizing drugs.

During this treatment, addicted people stop taking opiates and they allow their bodies to adjust to living without drugs. The individual will go through withdrawal symptoms. More about withdrawals and the symptoms you can expect, in the section below.

These opioid withdrawal symptoms continue for about 5 to 10 days in most of the cases. Though these symptoms are uncomfortable, they do not pose any substantial threat to the recovering addict. Opiate withdrawal is an important step in detoxification process but when individuals detox in a treatment or medical setting, many withdrawal symptoms can be subverted or at the least controlled by the use of rest, medication and many other methods of care and treatment.

Over-the-Counter Cures

Getting through pains, chills, fever, and aches is what overcoming opiate addiction is about. Ibuprofen, Tylenol and some of the other "non-addictive" pain alleviating agents could help in

46

easing some of your discomforts.

Taper Technique

This technique slowly and gradually reduces the amounts of dosage over time. This approach is helpful in reducing the withdrawal effects as the body would only have to adapt to minor reductions. Only can this be helpful if you stick to the plan and do not cheat i.e. do not get back to using drugs again.

Buprenorphine

Buprenorphine is used to treat opiate addictions as one of the therapies of opiate-replacement. This medication mimics the outcomes of opiates, but it does not pose a higher addiction risk. Buprenorphine could also be given by physicians as they have the authority to prescribe it.

Changes in Daily Routine

Most often the addiction of opiate spawns a lifestyle of its own. Habits or routines, like utilizing opiates before going to bed (i.e. sleep) or using them before going to work will have to be replaced with some healthy alternatives. Making a plan ahead of time could help.

Attending Support Groups

Support groups provide a source of support, guidance and camaraderie when trying to overcome opiate addiction. The group members in the support group share their experiences and extend their advice on the process of recovery and also cope during the hard times. There is no one to criticize which makes people comfortable. Support groups also help overcoming the depression that is caused as a result of sitting alone. However some connections at these groups can result in going back to your old ways, so make sure you pick the right people to be around.

Psychotherapy

Psychological addiction should be equally treated like the physical addiction. Psychotherapy treatment helps addicts recover through the forces that drive them to use opiates. This is also known as a behavioral treatment which involves an intensive therapy through talk. Through this procedure, people build up positive self-concepts.

Residential Treatment Programs

For people who have been relying on opiates since a long time require intense drug treatments. Comprehensive and structured care is provided by residential treatment programs and they are designed for helping the users to abstain from opiates for a long-term period until the person will no longer crave the drug.

"Residential opiate addiction treatment centers" provide an extensive range of specialized services and treatments that are designed especially to help people in overcoming their opiate addiction and helping them live a life free of drugs. These centers provide people the required group supports, ongoing psychotherapies, and medical care as effective methods for their opiate addiction treatment. Also, these centers closely supervise the people and give them ongoing care so they can resist the cravings (these come with the withdrawal).

Those who are in the recovery process have a higher potential of an overdose for them preventing relapse is very important to avoid the likelihood of an overdose. These centers use intensive treatment approaches which reduce the chances of a relapse.

"Residential opiate addiction treatment centers" offer the recovering addicts with a complete 24-hour access to therapists and counselors, who are

51

specialized in dealing with issues of opiate addiction.

Outpatient Treatment Programs

People who have completed their residential program could gain from ongoing treatments that are offered through outpatient programs. Though these programs are less restrictive, they help the addicts in staying engaged during the recovery process and develop skills required to cope with everyday life.

Outpatient programs offer support and help to people while allowing them to stay at home. This treatment does not require residential care or hospitalization. The decision of choosing outpatient treatment depends entirely on the severity of the problem.

Different stages of "outpatient treatment" used to treat opiate addiction include counseling, detoxification, long-term support, and aftercare. People with severe opiate addictions should not opt for outpatient treatments.

Individual Treatment Needs

It is important that a person receives the right treatment or else no amount of work or effort will help them in overcoming opiate addiction.

This case is particularly for long-term users of opiate. The first and most important step is to understand what kind of treatment will help you.

Each of the above-mentioned methods of treatment provides individuals with some medical support or monitoring, therapy and counseling, detox and aftercare. Some of these programs are longer as compared to the others. In order to make the opiate addiction treatments effective and safe, researchers propose that the programs should be of 90 days at least, and in severe cases they can be longer too.

Research has shown that it takes about 90 days in order to effectively break the habit and to bring changes in the behavior. For some people, it might take longer to overcome their addiction of opiate.

Chapter 6: Your Support System & Getting Real

Once you have had enough, and are no longer wanting to chase that elusive "high", **and really ready to make a change**, you are going to need support. You are going to need to tell people of your plan. This SHOULD NOT be your little kept secret. If your addiction has been a secret then this is the time for you to tell everyone of it.

The reason you need to tell people is not because you need them to know you have been taking painkillers just to get through each day. It's not because you need to be accountable for what you have been doing. The reason you need to tell people is because you need to be accountable for what you are going to do. You need to let as many people as you can, in on your venture of quitting opiates.

We're going to use a bit of psychology here. The more who know of your plan to quit taking opiates, the more ashamed and embarrassed you will feel if your plan fails. That is exactly what you want. The more embarrassed you might be of failure, the less likely the chances of failure.

Most people will be happier that you are quitting, than they will be upset at what you have been doing. You will know whom you can trust and whom you can't. You know which people will be the most helpful to you.

In fact, the most helpful people are the ones who will tell you that you can do it. If you have friends or family members that you have told this to before, who have seen you fail and now they don't believe you anymore, then these are not the people you should tell.

Avoid telling them until you have some time of sobriety in. The last thing you need is to hear people telling you that you can't or won't do it.

Tell the right people – the people who will be supportive of you. Tell the people who will be excited for you and whom will show it on their faces. Tell the people who are going to cheer you on. Tell the people who are not afraid to ask you how your sobriety is going later. In fact, ask them to ask you about your sobriety later.

You know who these people are. Tell as many of these people of your upcoming sobriety as you possibly can and avoid telling the naysayers, until later. Believe me, after you do this, you will try all the more to make it happen for you due to embarrassment of failure.

Keep in mind that I only use the word **failure** for lack of better word. I could use the word unsuccessful, however, **unsuccessful** doesn't quite have the stigma that it needs in order to make this part of the process work. But anytime that you don't find success it is never **failure**. It is a learning process that you can look back on and evaluate so as to not make the same mistakes the next time.

Now getting back to telling the world of your upcoming endeavor. If you don't want to tell people, here is another question to ask yourself. **What is the real reason I don't want people to know?** Is it because you are embarrassed or ashamed? Or is it because somewhere in the back of your mind, you are hoping that this does fail so that you can go right back to using?

To some, this question may sound ridiculous. But to many, it is an honest question that really needs to be answered. Many people want to quit, but they are so afraid of the unknown that they will subconsciously sabotage their own success. They cannot see the wonderful, life changing possibilities that lay before them. Are you one of those people? If so, the more you recognize this fact, the easier it will be to get over these negative thoughts.

Chapter 7: Choices for Detoxing

There are a few ways to go about this. You can quit cold turkey, you can taper off of the meds, and then there's Naltrexone, Suboxone and Methadone.

Cold Turkey:

If you are a heavy user, then tapering off of the meds is much less intimidating and the withdrawals are much easier to get through. With that being said, this can still hard to do even when tapering and even though the withdrawals are not as severe as going cold turkey, they will last longer. When you go cold turkey, the withdrawals can be pretty brutal. Well to be honest, they can be very brutal.

Taper Off The Meds:

How is your pain and sickness threshold? If you are one of those people who get sick and take it well, then maybe going cold turkey is right for you. You will detox much quicker and be done and ready to begin your new life. Or, are you one of those people who whine and moan and cry when you are sick (like me)? If that's the case, then tapering off may be the way to go. You need to decide which is right for. Know that these recommendations are not set in stone. They are merely suggestive, and only that. You are the only one who can make the decision on what is right for you.

Medications That Can Beat Opioid Addiction

If you are ready for treating your addiction then the following medications can help. But always consult a professional before using these.

- Revia (naltrexone)

- Suboxone or Subutex (buprenorphine)

- Methadone

Overcoming opiate addiction requires willpower. Counseling and medication can improve chances of success.

With the invention of new drugs like naltrexone and buprenorphine (sometimes they are combined with naloxone) and therapies such as using Methadone with 12-step programs, there has been success in helping thousands of people to recover from opiate addiction.

One of the standard treatments for treating opiate addiction requires Methadone. This is an oral long-acting opioid which helps in keeping withdrawal, relapse and cravings under control. Methadone is helpful for opiate addicts as it rehabilitates them and prevents the symptoms of withdrawal which can motivate to continue using drugs.

Naltrexone and naloxone are medications which oppose opioid receptors; this means that they can curtail the opiate urge by blocking the receptors of opiate so that when opiates are taken, they are unable to produce gratifying effects. The blockers alone sometimes are helpful for addicts who are highly propelled to quit. Also, scientists are preparing a durable version of naltrexone which would be required to be taken only once in a month.

Suboxone is another medication that can be used for detoxing and withdrawing from opiates. This medicine is a combination of buprenorphine (which is a mild opiate) and naloxone. Naloxone is a medication which reverses opiate's effects if it is taken intravenously.

Although Suboxone and Methadone are both used to treat opiate addiction, they are completely different. Methadone is much stronger than Suboxone because it is a full opiate that initiates a physiological response, whereas Suboxone is only partial. Because Methadone is so strong, it is not typically used for patients with less severe addictions. When this drug is given to a patient who has a light to moderate addiction, it can come with a severe side effect because the Methadone is so much stronger than the amount of opiates they were already taking. Doctors have been known to do this, unaware of this fact or consequences.

Methadone is much more addictive than Suboxone because it doesn't have a ceiling on its "high" effect. The more you take, the higher you get. There is a limit on how high you can get when taking Suboxone, no matter how much of it you take. That is why the withdrawals for this drug are much easier to handle than Methadone, and less addictive.

Because Suboxone is a mellower substitute for opiates, it is a drug that can be prescribed and then brought home by the patient. When treated with Methadone, a patient must visit the clinic daily to receive their daily doses. They are not allowed to bring it home with them because of a high risk of fatal overdose. However, further on in your treatment most Methadone clinics will allow take-home doses.

Suboxones' withdrawals are much easier to handle than Methadone. I personally haven't taken either of them, and I am so glad that I didn't have to. I have noticed that many of the people who are on Methadone are upping their doses and not lowering them. Methadone is an addiction that is even harder to break than what you may be doing now. Methadone is used to avoid withdrawals, and it works very well. But what happens when it's time to quit Methadone? The withdrawals are far worse than they would be coming off pain pills today. Methadone does work, and it may be something for you to look into if your addiction is severe. Just know that if you start it, you may not come off of it for years, many years.

Although I believe that Methadone is not a good choice, that doesn't mean that it's not right for everyone. It is harder to get off of than the pain pills you are taking and you would be on Methadone for quite some time. But to many people, the main goal is to get off of the opiates no matter what it takes. I believe by using a replacement therapy, you could be putting yourself right back into the same situation you are in, but for some people, it may be the only hope for recovery from opiates.

Chapter 8: Getting Ready for Detox

When you are getting ready for the big day, there are several things you will need to do. Your detox can take anywhere between five to eight days, give or take a day. Trust me, you will not want to do anything but lay around your house for most of this time, so taking some time off work in advance is a smart thing to do. If you don't, you can expect to have a lot call in sick days ahead of you. It's better to be prepared. This will be one less worry. If you have made the decision to taper off the drug, then you might not have to take the time off depending on how quick and extreme your taper is. If you are going to taper off slowly, you might be okay. But if you are planning on tapering off quickly, let's say, in a about a week, then you may need the time off as well.

Tell your doctor about your plan. Many people won't want to do this either because they want to ensure that they will still be able to get their meds later if plans change. If this is the case, then again, you need to take a serious look at exactly how serious you are. You could use your doctor's help. He will probably recommend and help you with a taper plan. If that is not what you want then ask him to give you some kind of muscle relaxer or anxiety medication. These medications won't make it all better or make the pain go away, but they will make it a bit easier to get through the next week. I would suggest using these medications whether you are going cold turkey or tapering. Either way you decide to do this, it's not going to be easy.

Some would say that using these medications is not a good idea because of the chance of forming a new addiction. If you go about it the right way, you will lower your chances of this happening. This is where your friends and family come in. You need to find a really close friend or relative who will be willing to assist you. Preferably your friend will be able to stay with you for a while during your detox, especially if you have children at home. If this isn't a possibility you need to at least be able to get in touch with this person every day while you're detoxing. When you get the medications from your doctor, give them to your new assistant. You will decide on a certain amount of this medication per day, and your friend will give you exactly that dose, and no more.

Try this out for a day, and if you need to up the dose and the amount in the prescription permits, then by all means, up the dose. Make sure your friend understands this before you give up the medication for them to hold. Your doctor will have a better insight on how much of this medication you should take, but sometimes doctors underestimate the severity of the withdrawals and give you as little as possible. But some is always better than none.

Your doctor may not be comfortable giving you a muscle relaxer or anxiety med. If not, ask him about Gabapentin, also known as Neurontin. This is a nerve medication that is used for epilepsy and nerve pain. When I slipped my disc I was given gabapentin. But I never took it because I had something much better. I had my Percocet.

I wish I could go back in time. I had bottles and bottles of it stacked under my bathroom sink. I got them from my doctor for years along with the Percocet. I saved them in case I ever hurt my back again and didn't have any Percocet. Little did I know at the time, that supposedly it works wonders for withdrawal symptoms too. Although there have been a small number of people who have become addicted to it, those are very unusual and rare cases as it doesn't give a euphoric feeling. It's not a narcotic. Your doctor may be happy as a clam to prescribe this one to you.

Gabapentin has been known to sometimes cure your withdrawals almost completely. This could be the miracle drug that all pain killer addicts have been searching for. If your doctor does give them to you, try it out for a day before your actual quit day. See if it works before you take time off work. You may not even need it. Now getting back to your detox in case the Gabapentin doesn't work for you as well as it does for others, or you simply can't get your hands on it.

Set up your home to be as comfortable as possible. Try and make sure that it is clean when you begin your detox. Make one big trip to the grocery store. Stock up on canned and frozen foods. You may want to get some fresh fruit and vegetables you can eat raw as well. Make sure you get plenty of things you can whip up quickly. You won't be very hungry, but you are still going to need to eat. The more food you have in your home, the more likely you are to eat something. If you're not hungry and you are trying to force yourself to eat, there is nothing worse than searching an empty refrigerator. Like I said before, once the detox starts, you won't want to do much, including cleaning, cooking and shopping.

Stock up on lots of movies on Netflix or another provider. Comedies are always best for situations like this because they are better at distracting you. I don't recommend reading books even if you are a reader. Chances are high that you won't even be able to pay much attention to the movies for the first few days let alone concentrate on a book.

This all sounds scary, I know. But remember, you are getting ready for your new beginning. It's all very worth it. I know because I've done it.

Chapter 9: Withdrawal Symptoms

Withdrawals are most commonly compared to flu like symptoms with people coming off pain pills and opioid addictions. However this not just any flu. It may be the worst flu you've ever had.

If your addiction is less severe, you'll probably only experience a few of these symptoms, however, if your addiction is heavy, your withdrawals will match the severity.

Here is what you can expect.

- Muscle and joint aches

- Insomnia (pain pills numb the feeling of being tired so you probably haven't felt truly tired in a while. Because of this, your tiredness will feel more severe)

- Nightmares (when you do sleep)

- Restless legs (temporary Restless Leg Syndrome)

- Diarrhea

- Hot and cold sweats

- The feeling of creepy crawlies under the skin (like Restless Leg Syndrome for the whole body)

- The shakes

- Exhaustion

- Depression

- Anxiety

- Loss of hunger

- Yawning

- Rapid heart beat

- Watering eyes and nose

- Goose bumps

- Pupil Dilation

- Sudden muscle jerks

- Back Pain

- Nausea and vomiting

- Lowered immune system (many people get a lowered immune system, which leads to rashes, acne breakouts, colds and infections)

- Hypnic or Hypnagogic jerk – Some people have dreams as if they are falling and have just hit the ground (this is how most people describe it). This causes a body jerk, which wakes them right away. Not everyone gets this, but it can be scary if you don't know what it is. This should only happen right before falling into REM sleep

Coping & Withdrawal Symptoms

If you are an opiate addict and want to get clean, then the only way is to stop taking these drugs. Sounds simple enough however we know it isn't. See, when you stop taking drugs, you will have to face withdrawal symptoms, as your body is used to them. Many addicts keep taking opiates to avoid these symptoms. The process of withdrawal is inevitable. Nothing is impossible; all you require is willpower and determination.

Home remedies for coping with withdrawal symptoms

People who are dependent on opiates, their bodies get used to them. The bodies develop tolerance to many different side effects of drugs, such as constipation and dryness. A strong reaction might be caused when these people stop taking opiates.

If you ever think about or are already thinking about going through withdrawal all by yourself, you will have to prepare yourself. Try tapering off opiates slowly before you stop using them completely, this will limit the withdrawal intensity. Nonetheless, due to the addiction's compulsive nature, almost all the people find it difficult to gradually reduce a number of opiates they take thus, they return back to their addiction.

Dehydration due to diarrhea and vomiting (withdrawal symptoms) is common which could result in serious health complications. Most of the people, due to dehydration, end up being in the hospital. During withdrawal, it is important to drink enough of hydrating fluids. Electrolyte solutions, like Pedialyte, might help in keeping you hydrated.

Over-the-Counter Help

Usage of right doses of over-the-counter medications could help. For diarrhea, take loperamide (Imodium). If you feel nauseated, try taking medications like dimenhydrinate (Dramamine) or meclizine (Bonine or Antivert). You can also take antihistamines like Benadryl. Pains and aches that appear unexpectedly and suddenly anywhere could be treated with NSAIDS like ibuprofen (Motrin, Advil) or acetaminophen (Tylenol).

Withdrawal symptoms could last for a few days or a few weeks. When taking medications for withdrawal symptoms, be very careful and stick to the recommended dose. If you think the regular dose is not making you feel better, then discuss the problem with your doctor.

Stay safe and comfortable

When going through withdrawal try staying comfortable. Keep yourself busy with books, movies or any other distraction. Make sure to have extra sheets, soft blankets, and a fan. Due to excess sweating you might have to change your bedding.

Make sure to tell about your withdrawal attempt to your family members or friends. You always need someone to keep a check on you. Be very vigilant of anecdotal stories and recipes described on different online forums. They have not been rigorously tested for efficacy and safety.

It is extremely important to keep yourself and your mind engaged and occupied. Do things that you enjoy in order to increase endorphins of your body. This can ameliorate the chances of long-term success.

Treating withdrawal

Some of the treatment methods could decrease the severity and length of the symptoms in order to make the opiate withdrawal process easy. Your doctor might suggest the following medications:

- Clonidine hydrochloride for treating common symptoms

- Naloxone for reducing the occurrence of symptoms

- Naltrexone for treating and reversing a heroin overdose

- Anesthesia for a speedy detoxification

Doctors also prescribe buprenorphine to keep people from relapsing after detox. Sometimes during the treatment, Buprenorphine is combined with naloxone. In cases of severe Methadone addiction, physicians might ask you to take the drug and then step by step decrease the dosage over time in order to reduce the dependence naturally.

Chapter 10:
How to Stay Clean

In order to stay off of pain pills, you are going to have to create a new environment. This doesn't mean that you have to weed out (no pun intended) your loved ones and all your friends or move away. Most people aren't in a position to do such things. Changing your environment can mean simply changing your way of living.

You can change many things in your life to make it feel different. Take another route to work every day. Change your hairstyle and your wardrobe. Change the furniture around in your home. You want to be able to look around and see things differently.

Remember, everything in your life as it is, is a trigger. You want to feel like a new person in every way. Doing these small, simple things can help you feel different. You will still be you, just a better, new you. It will still be your life and triggers will still be there. But they will be camouflaged.

Most people with addictions must replace their addiction with a new one. I would like to use the words "All people" but there is always an exception to everything. A compulsive behavior is already settled into the brain and it can't be removed without serious therapy. You are no different. You may not be able to find a replacement right away. But the longer you go, the more you may notice that you still have a strong want for the drug. This will not go away for quite some time if your addiction was moderate to severe. You will find that replacing the addiction will make it easier.

A new "addiction" doesn't mean a new drug. Find new activities and hobbies to replace it with. I call this a new "addiction" because it is usually something that people completely immerse themselves in. Many people replace their addictions with exercise or community engagement. Some replace it with arts and crafts. My new addiction is writing books. It's healthy as an outlet for me as is running.

Associating yourself with new people can help you find new activities to help keep you busy, and keep your compulsive behavior at bay. It has been said that social engagement can help people suffering as isolation is something that makes us repeat the cycle. When you associate yourself with new people, you will find yourself doing new things and avoiding old triggers. When meeting new people, try and find someone who understands your situation. It is always a wise idea to get involved with people who have been through what you are going through. You need as many supportive people as possible in your life.

People who understand you are important, however, the last thing you want to do is get yourself involved with people who are also new to recovery themselves. Associating with them online, over the phone or in a support group is one thing. There is no avoiding that unless you are planning on avoiding support groups all together, which I personally don't recommend. You will need all the support you can get. However, having newly recoveries privately close to you is different. It may take months or even years until you are ready for that.

I had a cousin who went to a recovery center for alcohol. When he got out, he kept in contact with many of the people he met in the recovery center. A few of them were in there for cocaine, which my cousin was also an addict to at one time. You can probably see where this is leading.

Needless to say, when my cousin got out, he didn't only relapse on his drinking, but he also began doing cocaine again because he was in such close contact to so many people who were doing it.

This is why I strongly encourage you to keep newly recovering addicts out of your personal life. People who have been in recovery for at least a year should be your ideal candidates. It really is treading dangerous waters to add unstable people to your life when you are still so vulnerable yourself.

There may be people already in your life that are also addicts. They might be simply acquaintances or they could be people very close to you. If they are just acquaintances it should be fairly easy to stay away from them. Not necessarily because you can't trust them, but most likely, it's yourself that you might not be able to trust. You might feel great. You might feel as strong as an ox. Unfortunately, you won't realize exactly how strong or weak you really are until you are around people who have, or are able to get you the goods.

Why take that chance after you have worked so hard?

Sometimes, such as if it's a spouse with the addiction, then you can't get away from it. Your spouse is most likely not going anywhere. But if you have made the decision to change your life no matter what your spouse chooses to do, then you need to try and find ways to be away from them as often as you can when they are using. Whether that be going out with healthy friends, or shutting yourself in another room and reading.

Unfortunately if you are involved with someone who is using and is not planning on quitting, statistics are very high that the relationship will fail. This is not to say that failure is inevitable. It's not. You may have to seek counseling for this kind of situation. But know that it is possible to make it work if enough effort is put into it.

If your partner doesn't want to quit, you can't force them. Don't wait around for someone to quit with you. It doesn't work that way. There are many times when couples want to quit an addiction.

The problem is, those moments come and go at different times for each person in the relationship. It is not common that the two of you will be on the same page at the same time. Take care of yourself and never mind what the other is doing. This goes for good friends as well.

During the recovery process you are going to have to get very comfortable with positive self-talk (affirmations). You will still need constant reassurance and you won't always be around other people to give it to you. Train yourself to lift yourself up, not only on a daily basis, but very often throughout each day. Start from the moment you wake up and continue until you go to bed every night. Stand in front of a mirror and say, "I am healthy, I am strong, and I am happy." Have you ever heard the saying, "they believe their own lies"? Even if you don't feel what you are saying is true at the time, the more you tell yourself how awesome you are, the more you begin to believe it.

You are awesome. You need to know that too.

When you are using self-talk, you don't want to mention your drug abuse. Only use positive affirmations. Using your addiction in your affirmations is counterproductive. It will just remind you of your history. You want to look forward, not back. Instead of saying, "I am so happy I don't take pills anymore," say, "I am so happy that I am mentally and physically healthy," or, "I am so happy for my new life."

Being thankful for each and every day of your sobriety is a must. It doesn't matter who you thank. Whether you are thankful to God, the universe, your friends and family or yourself, just be thankful. Like your affirmations, you should try and feel thankful often throughout your days. You can even combine your thanks and affirmations, like I did above. As you are reminding yourself how awesome you are, you can be thankful that you are as awesome as you are. The more thankful you are

about every positive thing in your life,
the more of those positive things you will
get.

Goals Can Make A Difference

These are all things that sound obvious and simple, and they are. But they are of the upmost importance as well. They go hand and hand with the success of your long-term sobriety. You can't have one without the other. It's as simple as that. So take it seriously and train yourself well.

Goals are also very simple but very important. Without goals, how can we achieve anything?

Before your detox, you should sit down and write out some short-term goals. Write down how you want your detox to go and how long it will take for you to be up and out of your house again. Write down a list of the people you might contact about your plan and what you will say. Write down a goal to clean one room a day while you are detoxing if you would like.

This list will be mostly a practice list, yet you should still be attempting to achieve these goals too. When you are finished with your detox, you should write another list of your long-term goals on what you would like to do with your new found life. Goals mean you have something to work toward. You have a lot of work ahead of you. Make it worth something.

While we are on the subject of lists, writing a list of positive things your recovery will bring you is a great daily reminder. You should do this before you begin your detox. I personally wouldn't make this a pros and cons list of taking painkillers. That is another way to bring up your past drug use. Instead, just make it a pros list. Think of your future and how you want it to be. Then write a list on how being Sober will help you. For instance: Being sober will help me save money. Being sober will help my relationships with my family members.

Of course when you write these lists, there is no way to write them without thinking about the negative affects the drugs have caused in your life. That is okay. You have to think about them. The point is to think about them momentarily, simply in order to find positive things to compare them to. You don't want to dwell, and reminding yourself of your past can cause you to dwell on it. So think of negative things that your drug use has done. Then, find positive opposites and write them down on your lists. After your list is complete, let those negative thoughts go and focus on your lists

What to do if you relapse

Relapse is very common among the addicts and it should be expected. It happens more often than not. You are addicted to something really strong and you may need a few times to "heal".

See, during the recovery process, there is always a risk for relapse. As the withdrawal process is painful, individuals at some point quit and get back to taking opiates. Relapse is one of the stages of opiate addiction treatment.

Some people begin their recovery process from where they left off after relapsing.

Opiate addictions leave long-lasting impressions on the chemical functions and processes of the brain. These effects then make the recovering addict capable of relapsing for the years to come.

Relapse causes vary from person to person:

- Daily life pressures

- Co-occurring conditions, like anxiety disorders and depression

- Lack of social support

- Interpersonal conflicts

- Poor coping skills

- Lack of dedication in recovery process

Starting again with the opiate addiction treatment after you have relapsed could help you in identifying your problem areas and taking different steps in order to strengthen your recovery process.

After a relapse treat yourself by talking with counsellors and using psychotherapy. It will take a few weeks and it will help ensure that you do not relapse again.

Coping with Prescription Drug Abuse

Conquering prescription drug abuse is a very challenging task. It can trigger a lot of stress in the person trying to overcome it, as well as create difficulties for his/her family. This ordeal will require much support from friends, family, and even groups. You can approach the following for support during your treatment of prescription drug abuse:

- Trusted circle of family and friends

- Groups similar to Alcoholics Anonymous that have programs that you can adapt or follow

- Religious organizations or church groups that aim to assist and help those who are on their way to recovery

- School guidance counselors

- Support groups in your local community (try to avoid online forums if possible, as a lot of misinformation can be found online)

- Company assistance programs for employees, such as counseling for those who have drug abuse problems

Do not be embarrassed to solicit help from your friends and family members. The main thing that keeps us back is the fear of being judged, or that family and friends may get angry at you.

However, looking at the bigger picture, people who genuinely care for you will help you out and accept you for who you are. They will go the extra mile to help you overcome a prescription drug addiction and will believe in you even when you may struggle to believe in yourself.

Helping a family member or friend

It may not be easy to confront another person about prescription drug abuse, especially if he or she is a close family member or a good friend. You will commonly encounter denial or anger. These are expected reactions and it is also normal that you will be hesitant about damaging your relationship. But it is important to help the family member or friend who is abusing prescription drugs before things get out of hand.

You have to be patient and understanding towards the person.

Make sure that you make your concern and care known to that person. Encourage honesty and be there to help, if needed. If the person trusts you enough and has the internal motivation, then he/she will most likely take action on their situation. However, if the case worsens, then it is best to approach an expert.

It is not easy to help family members or close friends dealing with prescription drug abuse. They will usually not be willing to seek medical help despite them needing it badly. They will not see, at least at first, that what they are doing is harmful to them and the people around them.

Focus on telling the person about the positives that they will experience from overcoming their problem. Point out the negative affects in their life, but stay away from harping on the issue to the point that they will become angry at your presence in their life.

Intervention

Intervention is a process that is carefully planned out. This involves family or friends, or both, as well as concerned people who care about the person that is going through prescription drug abuse. To have an effective intervention, it is important to consult an intervention specialist, addiction specialist, and a mental health therapist. They will all work together to help the person understand about the dangers of prescription drug abuse and ask them to agree to undergo treatment.

Preventing Prescription Drug Abuse

When you are prescribed a drug, it does not mean that you are at a high risk of drug abuse or addiction. Drug abuse does not happen often among those who are using sedatives, stimulants, or painkillers for their medical condition. But if you are taking a medication that is commonly abused, then here are some helpful tips for you to lower your risk of drug abuse:

See to it that you are getting the correct medication for your condition. When you visit your physician or health care provider, it is important that you are diagnosed correctly and that your symptoms are understood. Let your doctor know about all the other prescriptions that you have and any other medication that you are taking, such as over-the-counter drugs, herbs, and other supplements. You can also ask your physician if there is an alternative drug that you can take that has a lesser potential for addiction.

Make sure that you follow the directions carefully. Only use the medication based on the way that it was prescribed to you. Do not stop taking the medication unless you are otherwise instructed. Never change the dosage on your own without consulting your physician. If you have a painkiller that does not seem to relieve your pain, then do not take in more than the required dosage. Ask your doctor what you can do about it and wait for his/her prescription.

Talk with your doctor every now and then to make sure that the medication you are taking is working and that you are using the correct dosage that was prescribed to you.

It is important that you know the effects of the medication that you are taking before you consume it. Ask the physician or pharmacist about any effects of the drug, so that you will be familiar with what to expect.

When ordering medications online, make sure to look for a reliable pharmacy. There are online pharmacies that are selling counterfeit drugs that can be dangerous to your health. Make sure that you only order from a legit online pharmacy.

Chapter 11: Conclusion

I have been there. My cousin became one of the statistics. Things can look hopeless. But with understanding, some work, it can truly become better for you, me and all of America (and any other country with an opioid crisis) if we take action now.

We were seeing the quiet mutterings of an opioid epidemic coming, and now brazenly showing up, on front pages everywhere, front of mind, in our own small towns and cities. We must do something to put an end to it, and heal.

America can do this. America can heal.
We all need to heal together.

I have worked hard creating the best "to-the-point" guide I know about

America's opioid epidemic, and how we got here, what can be done, and most importantly, how we can heal from it. We are truly in an opioid crisis and need to take back control and show how can overcome America's dependence on prescription and drug addiction.

It's now up to You, to pull out this book what you can take from it and what resonates with you. Take those pieces and implement them.

Lastly, if you found this book beneficial, then I'd like to ask you for a favor. Would you be so kind to leave a review for this book on Amazon? It would be very much appreciated!

Thank you!

D.W. Graeme

Made in the USA
Lexington, KY
26 January 2018